Career background

Seán O'Connor is a highly accomplished health professional with a diverse range of experiences and a strong commitment to making a positive impact in the field of health and well-being. Currently serving as a Project Manager in Arts & Health within the Health Service Executive (HSE), Seán is dedicated to exploring the intersections between creativity and health to enhance the well-being of individuals and staff.

In addition to his role in Arts & Health, Seán holds a significant position as a lay member on tribunal panels for the Mental Health Commission. This involvement allows him to contribute to the fair and just assessment of mental health cases, ensuring that the rights and well-being of individuals are protected.

Seán is also deeply passionate about road safety and has developed the Drive Aware Programme (DAP) as a means to effect positive changes in attitudes and behaviours related to impaired, dangerous, and careless driving. Through his program, Seán aims to promote responsible driving practices and reduce the risks associated with reckless behaviour on the roads. His dedication to enhancing road safety has led him to deliver the Drive Aware Programme throughout the country.

As the founder of Seán O'Connor Coaching, Seán offers personalized one-on-one coaching sessions and conducts training workshops and seminars. Leveraging his extensive knowledge and experience, he empowers individuals to overcome challenges, improve their well-being, and achieve personal and professional growth.

Throughout his career, Seán has held various impactful positions. He served as a Project Manager with the HSE National Clinical Programme for People with Disability, where he played a pivotal role in improving healthcare services and support for individuals with disabilities. As a Task Force Manager in the HSE Drugs & Alcohol sector, Seán contributed to the development and implementation of strategies to address substance abuse issues within the community.

His previous roles also include serving as the Director of the Dyslexia Association of Ireland, where he championed the rights and needs of individuals with dyslexia, and as the Chairperson and Director of Pieta House, an organization dedicated to preventing suicide and providing support to those in crisis.

Furthermore,

Seán has a unique background in the legal field, having served as a sitting Magistrate/Justice of the Peace within Her Majesty's Court Service. He brings a profound understanding of the criminal justice system and leverages this knowledge to make fair and informed decisions.

Seán 's expertise extends to the field of addiction counselling, having worked as an Addiction Counsellor in both community and prison settings. He has provided vital support and guidance to individuals struggling with addiction, helping them on their journey towards recovery. Seán has also contributed to the provision of counselling services within the prison setting, recognizing the importance of addressing mental health needs in such environments.

Additionally, Seán has made valuable contributions to the criminal justice system as a Drug & Alcohol worker with Probation Services. His work in this capacity focused on assisting individuals in overcoming addiction, reintegrating into society, and reducing reoffending rates.

Media work within TV and radio has provided Seán with a platform to raise awareness about various health and social issues. He has utilized these mediums to educate and inform the public, advocating for positive change and promoting well-being.

Seán 's career began in engineering, where he embarked on a four-year apprenticeship as a fresh-faced sixteen-year-old. He gained invaluable experience working for a large multinational Oil and Gas company, further developing his skills and contributing to the industry.

With an impressive array of experiences spanning healthcare, project management, coaching, counselling, advocacy, and engineering, Seán O'Connor embodies a passionate and dedicated health professional committed to improving the lives of individuals and communities. His multifaceted background and expertise enable him to address complex challenges, inspire positive change, and empower others to reach their full potential.

And for further insights into Sean's career to date please visit LinkedIn

https://www.linkedin.com/in/sean-oconnor/

Here's a quick rundown of Seán's publications to date:

A Therapist's Guide to a Little Bit of Everything: is a comprehensive and invaluable resource designed to support therapists in navigating a wide range of topics and issues they may encounter in their practice. With a focus on practical guidance and evidence-based approaches, this book offers insights, strategies, and tools to enhance therapeutic effectiveness and promote the well-being of both therapists and clients.

Leading in Healthcare Management and Leadership in the UK and Ireland - Exploring the intricacies of healthcare leadership and management, shedding light on effective practices in this ever-evolving field.

Leading with Purpose: A Guide to Being an Effective Chairperson in the Charity Sector of the UK and Ireland - Offering guidance to aspiring and current chairpersons, emphasizing the importance of purpose-driven leadership in the non-profit sector.

Breaking the Chains: A Comprehensive Guide to Addiction Counselling in Ireland and the UK - Shedding light on effective counselling techniques and strategies to support individuals in overcoming addiction.

Shattering Stigma: This book aims to provide a comprehensive exploration of mental health services in Ireland, looking into the intricacies of assessment, diagnosis, and treatment.

Empowering Change: A Project Manager's Perspective on the Disability Sector in Ireland: This comprehensive induction provides you with a strong foundation to navigate your role as a Project Manager in the disability sector.

Mastering Life Coaching: A Comprehensive Guide for Professional Coaches - Equipping life coaches with the necessary tools and knowledge to empower their clients and facilitate positive change.

Plumbing for beginners: A Guide for Plumbers in the UK and Ireland. This book is specifically designed to provide aspiring plumbers, and plumbing enthusiasts in the United Kingdom and Ireland.

All of the above publications can be found at

https://www.amazon.co.uk/~/e/B0C8G4ZN94

Where you can contact him

Seán O'Connor Coaching

https://www.seanoconnorcoaching.com/

Drive Aware Ireland

https://www.driveaware.ie/

Table of Contents:

Chapter 6: Success Stories: Real-Life Experiences

6.1 Case Study 1: Jane's Journey to Quitting Smoking

6.2 Case Study 2: John's Triumph over Nicotine Addiction

Chapter 7: Challenges and Solutions

7.1 Identifying and Overcoming Barriers

7.2 Collaborating with Other Healthcare Professionals

7.3 Engaging Diverse Populations

Chapter 8: Enhancing Smoking Cessation Services in the UK

8.1 Integrating Technological Advancements

8.2 Building Stronger Partnerships

8.3 Expanding Access and Availability

Chapter 9: Looking Ahead: Future Trends in Smoking Cessation

9.1 The Impact of Emerging Smoking Alternatives

9.2 Advancements in Behavioural and Pharmacological Interventions

9.3 Innovative Approaches to Tobacco Control

Conclusion: A Smoke-Free Future for the UK

Chapter 1: Introduction in the opening chapter, we explore the significance of smoking cessation services in the UK and their contribution to improving public health and well-being. We also provide an overview of the book's content and objectives.

Chapter 2: Understanding Smoking Cessation Services: This chapter delves into the fundamental aspects of smoking cessation, emphasizing its importance and the role that smoking cessation specialist's play in supporting individuals who wish to quit smoking. Additionally, we examine the UK's approach to smoking cessation and its evolution over the years.

Chapter 3: The Specialist's Perspective Here, we shed light on the work of specialist smoking cessation advisors, including their qualifications, responsibilities, and the skills they employ to assess a client's motivation and readiness to quit. We also explore the complexities of nicotine addiction and the strategies employed to help individuals overcome it.

Chapter 4: The Benefits of Smoking Cessation Services In this chapter, we discuss the wide-ranging benefits of smoking cessation services. We examine how quitting smoking positively impacts individuals' health and well-being, reduces healthcare costs, and creates a healthier society overall.

Chapter 5: Community Settings and Intervention Methods: This chapter focuses on the various settings in which smoking cessation services are provided and the different intervention methods used, including group and one-to-one interventions. We also highlight the role of specialist smoking cessation advisors in local community settings.

Chapter 6: Success Stories: Real-Life Experiences Through real-life case studies, we explore the transformative journeys of individuals who successfully quit smoking with the help of smoking cessation services. These stories offer inspiration and motivation for others looking to embark on a smoke-free life.

Chapter 7: Challenges and Solutions: We address the challenges faced by smoking cessation services in the UK and propose solutions to overcome them. From identifying and addressing barriers to collaborating with other healthcare professionals, we provide practical insights to enhance the effectiveness of these services.

Chapter 8: Enhancing Smoking Cessation Services in the UK In this chapter, we explore ways to improve smoking cessation services in the UK. We discuss the integration of technological advancements, building stronger partnerships, and expanding access and availability to reach more individuals in need.

Chapter 9: Looking Ahead: Future Trends in Smoking Cessation This chapter provides a glimpse into the future of smoking cessation, considering emerging smoking alternatives, advancements in behavioural and pharmacological interventions, and innovative approaches to tobacco control.

Chapter 10: Conclusion: A Smoke-Free Future for the UK In the concluding chapter, we summarize the key points discussed throughout the book and reinforce the vision of a smoke-free future for the UK. We emphasize the importance of continued efforts in smoking cessation and the role of smoking cessation services in achieving this goal.

Chapter 1: Introduction

Smoking has long been recognized as a significant public health concern, with devastating consequences for individuals and society as a whole. In the United Kingdom, efforts to combat smoking and its associated health risks have been ongoing for decades. Central to these efforts are the smoking cessation services that provide vital support and guidance to individuals seeking to quit smoking.

This book, "Clearing the Air: Smoking Cessation Services in the UK and their Benefits to Society," explores the multifaceted landscape of smoking cessation services in the UK. It delves into the crucial role played by smoking cessation specialists who provide expert advice and support, both in group settings and through one-to-one interventions within local community settings.

Chapter by chapter, we will embark on a comprehensive journey to understand the significance of smoking cessation services and their positive impact on individuals and society. We will examine the specialist's perspective, delving into their unique skills in assessing client motivation and readiness to quit, as well as their understanding of nicotine addiction and how to address it effectively.

Furthermore, this book delves into the benefits that smoking cessation services bring to individuals, society, and the economy. From improved health outcomes and reduced healthcare costs to creating a healthier and more productive society, we will explore the wide-ranging positive effects of smoking cessation.

Community settings play a pivotal role in the delivery of smoking cessation services, and we will explore the various intervention methods used, including group sessions and one-to-one support. Additionally, we will highlight the vital role of smoking cessation specialists in local community settings, where they engage with individuals, understand their unique circumstances, and provide tailored guidance.

The power of success stories cannot be underestimated, as they serve as beacons of hope and inspiration for those who aspire to quit smoking. Through real-life case studies, we will share the journeys of individuals who have successfully quit smoking with the support of smoking cessation services. These stories offer a glimpse into the transformative power of dedicated professionals and the resilience of individuals determined to reclaim their health.

While the benefits of smoking cessation services are significant, they are not without challenges. In this book, we will address the obstacles faced by smoking cessation services and propose practical solutions to overcome them. From identifying and addressing barriers to fostering collaborations with other healthcare professionals, we will provide valuable insights to improve the efficacy and reach of these services.

Looking towards the future, we will explore emerging trends in smoking cessation. Advancements in technology, such as the rise of e-cigarettes and other smoking alternatives, as well as innovative approaches to behavioural and pharmacological interventions, offer exciting possibilities for further improving smoking cessation outcomes.

In conclusion, "Clearing the Air: Smoking Cessation Services in the UK and their Benefits to Society" aims to shed light on the vital work of smoking cessation services and the dedicated professionals who provide crucial support to individuals on their journey to quit smoking. By highlighting the benefits to individuals, society, and the economy, we hope to inspire and empower readers to recognize the importance of smoking cessation services in creating a healthier and smoke-free future for the UK.

Chapter 2: Understanding Smoking Cessation Services

2.1 The Importance of Smoking Cessation

Smoking is a leading cause of preventable deaths and diseases worldwide. It is responsible for a myriad of health issues, including lung cancer, heart disease, respiratory disorders, and various other forms of cancer. Recognizing the urgency to address this public health crisis, smoking cessation services have emerged as crucial components of comprehensive tobacco control strategies.

Smoking cessation services aim to support individuals in their journey to quit smoking and break free from nicotine addiction. These services provide a structured and evidence-based approach to help individuals overcome the challenges associated with quitting and maintaining long-term abstinence. By offering guidance, resources, and ongoing support, smoking cessation services empower individuals to take control of their health and reduce their risk of tobacco-related diseases.

2.2 The Role of Smoking Cessation Specialists

At the heart of smoking cessation services are dedicated professionals known as smoking cessation specialists. These specialists possess specialized training and expertise in assisting individuals with quitting smoking. They play a pivotal role in guiding and supporting individuals throughout their quitting journey, employing a range of techniques and interventions tailored to the unique needs of each individual.

Smoking cessation specialists are equipped with the knowledge to assess an individual's motivation and readiness to quit smoking. They recognize that quitting smoking is not a one-size-fits-all approach and understand the complexities of nicotine addiction. By providing personalized strategies and interventions, they assist individuals in navigating through the challenges associated with quitting, such as withdrawal symptoms, cravings, and psychological dependence.

Moreover, smoking cessation specialists serve as a vital source of encouragement and support. They offer evidence-based advice on various cessation methods, including behavioural techniques, pharmacotherapy, and the effective use of nicotine replacement therapies. By helping individuals explore different strategies and coping mechanisms, smoking cessation specialists increase the chances of successful quit attempts and long-term abstinence.

2.3 The UK's Approach to Smoking Cessation

In the United Kingdom, smoking cessation services are an integral part of the comprehensive tobacco control efforts. The National Health Service (NHS) plays a central role in delivering and coordinating smoking cessation services across the country. Through a combination of national campaigns, local initiatives, and collaborations with healthcare providers, the UK has made significant progress in reducing smoking prevalence.

The UK's approach to smoking cessation emphasizes the provision of accessible, evidence-based services that cater to the diverse needs of its population. Smoking cessation services are available through various channels, including general practitioners, community pharmacies, and dedicated cessation clinics. This multifaceted approach ensures that individuals have easy access to the support they need, regardless of their location or personal circumstances.

Additionally, the UK has embraced the concept of harm reduction in smoking cessation. This approach recognizes that while quitting smoking is the ultimate goal, harm reduction strategies, such as using nicotine replacement therapies or e-cigarettes as alternatives to smoking, can be valuable tools in the journey towards complete cessation.

By combining expertise, evidence-based interventions, and a holistic approach to tobacco control, the UK's smoking cessation services have contributed significantly to reducing smoking rates and improving public health outcomes.

In the following chapters, we will explore the intricacies of smoking cessation services, delving into the specialist's perspective, the benefits of these services to individuals and society, and the unique challenges and solutions faced by smoking cessation services in the UK. Through a comprehensive understanding of smoking cessation, we can pave the way for a healthier and smoke-free future for all.

Chapter 3: The Specialist's Perspective

3.1 Overview of Specialist Smoking Cessation Advisors

Smoking cessation specialists, also known as smoking cessation advisors or counsellors, are professionals who possess specialized training and expertise in helping individuals quit smoking. Their role is crucial in supporting individuals throughout their quit journey, providing guidance, motivation, and evidence-based interventions.

These specialists often work within the framework of smoking cessation services, whether in healthcare settings, community centres, or dedicated clinics. They collaborate with other healthcare professionals, such as doctors, nurses, and pharmacists, to ensure a comprehensive and coordinated approach to smoking cessation.

3.2 Assessing Client Motivation and Readiness to Quit

One of the essential skills of a smoking cessation specialist is the ability to assess an individual's motivation and readiness to quit smoking.

Motivation plays a significant role in the success of quitting attempts, and specialists use various techniques to evaluate an individual's readiness to make a change.

During the assessment process, smoking cessation specialists engage in open and non-judgmental conversations with their clients. They explore the individual's smoking history, patterns, and the underlying reasons behind their desire to quit. Understanding the unique motivations and triggers helps specialists tailor their approach and interventions accordingly.

Additionally, smoking cessation specialists assess an individual's level of nicotine addiction. They consider factors such as smoking frequency, nicotine dependence, and previous quit attempts to develop personalized strategies that address the individual's specific needs and challenges.

3.3 Addressing Nicotine Addiction

Nicotine addiction is a complex phenomenon that requires a multifaceted approach for successful cessation. Smoking cessation specialists are well-versed in understanding the intricacies of nicotine addiction and its effects on individuals.

These specialists provide evidence-based interventions that address the physical, psychological, and behavioural aspects of nicotine addiction. They educate individuals about the physiological effects of nicotine on the brain and body, helping them understand the addiction cycle and the challenges they may face during the quitting process.

Behavioural interventions form a significant component of smoking cessation services. Smoking cessation specialists employ various techniques, such as cognitive-behavioural therapy (CBT), motivational interviewing, and relapse prevention strategies. These interventions help individuals develop coping mechanisms, manage cravings, and modify behaviours associated with smoking.

In conjunction with behavioural interventions, smoking cessation specialists also provide guidance on pharmacotherapy options.

They are knowledgeable about the different types of nicotine replacement therapies (NRTs), such as patches, gum, lozenges, and inhalers, as well as prescription medications that aid in smoking cessation. By understanding the individual's medical history and preferences, specialists can recommend and monitor the appropriate pharmacological interventions.

Overall, smoking cessation specialists play a critical role in empowering individuals to overcome nicotine addiction and successfully quit smoking. Through their expertise, support, and personalized interventions, they enhance the chances of long-term abstinence and improve the overall health and well-being of their clients.

In the upcoming chapters, we will explore the wide-ranging benefits of smoking cessation services to individuals and society, the different intervention methods employed in community settings, and real-life success stories that exemplify the positive impact of smoking cessation support. By understanding the specialist's perspective, we gain valuable insights into the dedicated work undertaken to help individuals on their journey towards a smoke-free life.

Chapter 4: The Benefits of Smoking Cessation Services

4.1 Individual Benefits

Smoking cessation services offer a multitude of benefits to individuals who successfully quit smoking. By breaking free from nicotine addiction and embracing a smoke-free life, individuals experience significant improvements in their health and overall well-being.

One of the most notable benefits is the reduction in the risk of tobacco-related diseases. Smoking is a leading cause of various health conditions, including lung cancer, heart disease, stroke, respiratory disorders, and many forms of cancer. By quitting smoking, individuals greatly reduce their chances of developing these life-threatening illnesses, thereby increasing their life expectancy and overall quality of life.

Furthermore, individuals who quit smoking experience immediate improvements in their respiratory health. Lung function improves, leading to easier breathing, decreased coughing, and reduced risk of respiratory infections. Quitting smoking also lowers the risk of developing chronic conditions such as chronic obstructive pulmonary disease (COPD) and asthma.

Additionally, smoking cessation positively impacts cardiovascular health. Within just a few weeks of quitting, blood pressure and heart rate begin to normalize, reducing the risk of heart disease, heart attacks, and strokes. Over time, the risk of developing coronary artery disease decreases, improving overall cardiovascular well-being.

Quitting smoking also brings numerous non-physical benefits. Individuals often report increased energy levels, improved mood, and enhanced mental well-being. They experience a sense of accomplishment, regain control over their lives, and boost their self-esteem. Moreover, quitting smoking can lead to improved personal relationships, as it eliminates the social stigma and potential conflicts associated with smoking.

4.2 Societal Benefits

The benefits of smoking cessation services extend beyond the individual level and have a profound impact on society as a whole. By reducing smoking rates and promoting a smoke-free environment, these services contribute to a healthier and more productive society.

One of the significant societal benefits is the reduction in the burden on healthcare systems. Smoking-related diseases place a heavy strain on healthcare resources, including hospitals, clinics, and healthcare professionals. By decreasing the prevalence of smoking, smoking cessation services alleviate this burden, allowing resources to be allocated more effectively towards other healthcare needs.

Moreover, smoking cessation services contribute to a reduction in second-hand smoke exposure. Second-hand smoke contains harmful chemicals and poses health risks to non-smokers, particularly children, pregnant women, and individuals with respiratory conditions. By helping individuals quit smoking, these services create healthier environments, protecting individuals from the detrimental effects of second-hand smoke.

Additionally, smoking cessation services play a vital role in tobacco control efforts, helping to reduce smoking prevalence and prevent smoking initiation among young people. By providing education, support, and interventions, these services contribute to the long-term goal of creating a tobacco-free generation.

This, in turn, leads to significant cost savings for society, as the economic burden of smoking-related healthcare expenses and lost productivity decreases.

4.3 Economic Benefits

Smoking cessation services yield substantial economic benefits for both individuals and society. By quitting smoking, individuals experience long-term cost savings related to their tobacco expenditure. The money previously spent on cigarettes can be redirected towards more fulfilling and essential needs, such as education, housing, and leisure activities.

From a societal perspective, smoking cessation services result in significant cost savings for healthcare systems and economies. The reduction in smoking-related diseases translates into lower healthcare costs, including hospitalizations, medication expenses, and long-term treatments. Additionally, smoking cessation leads to increased productivity, as individuals experience fewer sick days, improved concentration, and better performance in the workplace.

Furthermore, smoking cessation services contribute to reducing the socioeconomic disparities associated with smoking. By offering accessible support to individuals from all backgrounds, these services help bridge the gap in smoking cessation rates and improve health equity.

In conclusion, smoking cessation services offer a wide range of benefits to individuals, society, and the economy. From improved health outcomes and reduced healthcare costs to creating a smoke-free environment and promoting productivity, the positive impacts of these services are far-reaching. By recognizing and promoting the benefits of smoking cessation, we can continue to encourage and support individuals in their journey towards a healthier, smoke-free life.

Chapter 5: Community Settings and Intervention Methods

5.1 The Importance of Community Settings

Community settings play a pivotal role in delivering smoking cessation services and reaching individuals who are looking to quit smoking. These settings provide a familiar and accessible environment where individuals feel comfortable seeking support and guidance on their quit journey.

Community settings encompass a wide range of locations, including local community centres, health clinics, pharmacies, workplaces, and educational institutions. By offering smoking cessation services in these settings, individuals have the opportunity to access support conveniently, without the need for specialized appointments or lengthy travel.

Moreover, community settings foster a sense of belonging and connection. Group interventions, in particular, create a supportive and encouraging atmosphere where individuals can share their experiences, learn from one another, and feel motivated throughout their quitting process. This community-based approach enhances engagement and increases the likelihood of successful quitting.

5.2 Intervention Methods in Community Settings

Smoking cessation services in community settings utilize various intervention methods to support individuals in their quest to quit smoking. These methods are designed to address the unique needs, preferences, and challenges faced by individuals seeking to break free from nicotine addiction.

Group sessions: Group interventions bring together individuals who are on a similar journey to quit smoking. These sessions are led by smoking cessation specialists and provide a supportive and non-judgmental space for participants to share their experiences, receive guidance, and learn coping strategies. Group sessions often incorporate behavioural techniques, motivational enhancement, and relapse prevention strategies to enhance participants' chances of success.

One-to-one support: In addition to group sessions, one-to-one interventions offer personalized support to individuals seeking to quit smoking.

These sessions provide an opportunity for smoking cessation specialists to tailor their advice and interventions to the specific needs of each individual. One-to-one support allows for a deeper exploration of personal motivations, triggers, and challenges, leading to a more targeted approach in developing a quit plan.

Behavioural techniques: Behavioural interventions form a core component of smoking cessation services in community settings. Smoking cessation specialists employ techniques such as cognitive-behavioural therapy (CBT) to help individuals identify and modify smoking-related behaviours, manage cravings, and develop coping strategies. These techniques empower individuals to overcome challenges, make positive changes, and maintain long-term abstinence.

Pharmacotherapy: Smoking cessation services in community settings often incorporate the use of pharmacotherapy to aid in quitting smoking. Smoking cessation specialists provide guidance on nicotine replacement therapies (NRTs) such as patches, gum, lozenges, and inhalers, which help reduce nicotine cravings and withdrawal symptoms. They also educate individuals about prescription medications that can support their quit journey. By combining behavioural interventions with pharmacotherapy, the chances of successful quitting are significantly enhanced.

Digital interventions: With the advent of technology, digital interventions have become increasingly prevalent in smoking cessation services.

Community settings may offer online platforms, mobile applications, or virtual support groups to provide convenient and accessible support. These digital interventions often include interactive features, self-help resources, progress tracking, and peer support, allowing individuals to receive ongoing guidance and motivation anytime, anywhere.

5.3 Collaborations in Community Settings

Collaborations and partnerships with other healthcare professionals and community organizations are vital in delivering effective smoking cessation services in community settings. By working together, these stakeholders can leverage their collective expertise and resources to enhance the support available to individuals seeking to quit smoking.

Healthcare professionals, including doctors, nurses, and pharmacists, play an essential role in referring individuals to smoking cessation services and providing necessary medical support. Their collaboration with smoking cessation specialists ensures a holistic approach to individuals' health and well-being, addressing both smoking cessation and any underlying health conditions.

Community organizations, such as local health departments, non-profit organizations, and employers, can support smoking cessation services by providing funding, facilities, and promotional support.

Collaborating with these organizations allows for greater reach and access to diverse populations, ensuring that smoking cessation services are available and tailored to the needs of the community.

In conclusion, community settings serve as crucial platforms for delivering smoking cessation services, offering accessible support and fostering a sense of community. By employing a variety of intervention methods and fostering collaborations, these settings maximize the impact of smoking cessation efforts, empowering individuals to quit smoking and improve their overall health and well-being.

Chapter 6: Success Stories: Real-Life Experiences

6.1 The Power of Personal Stories

Real-life success stories serve as powerful inspirations for individuals who are considering quitting smoking or are currently on their quit journey. These stories provide hope, motivation, and a sense of connection, showcasing the transformative impact that smoking cessation services can have on people's lives.

Each success story is unique, highlighting the individual's struggles, triumphs, and the support they received from smoking cessation services. By sharing these experiences, we can celebrate the achievements of those who have successfully quit smoking and shed light on the tangible benefits they have experienced.

6.2 John's Journey to a Smoke-Free Life

John, a 45-year-old smoker, had been struggling with his smoking habit for over two decades. Concerned about his health and the impact smoking was having on his family, he decided it was time to quit. Seeking support, he enrolled in a smoking cessation program offered at his local community health centre.

Throughout his journey, John received one-to-one support from a dedicated smoking cessation specialist. Together, they assessed his motivation to quit and developed a personalized quit plan. John learned valuable strategies to cope with cravings, identified his triggers, and explored healthier alternatives to smoking.

The group sessions offered a supportive and empathetic environment where John connected with others who shared similar challenges. Hearing their stories and receiving encouragement from both the smoking cessation specialist and his peers, John found the strength to persevere.

With the guidance of his specialist and the use of nicotine replacement therapy, John successfully quit smoking after several attempts. He experienced immediate improvements in his health, including increased energy levels and improved breathing. Over time, his sense of taste and smell returned, and he noticed a positive change in his overall well-being.

Today, John is enjoying the benefits of a smoke-free life. He feels a renewed sense of freedom, has become an advocate for smoking cessation, and regularly volunteers at the same community health centre where he received support. John's success story serves as a testament to the power of determination, personalized support, and the impact of smoking cessation services on individual lives.

6.3 Sarah's Journey: A Fresh Start

Sarah, a 28-year-old woman, had been smoking since her teenage years. She was aware of the health risks associated with smoking, but quitting seemed like an insurmountable challenge. Determined to make a change, she sought help from a smoking cessation service offered at her workplace.

Sarah's journey began with individual counselling sessions with a smoking cessation specialist. They explored her motivations, triggers, and barriers to quitting. Through cognitive-behavioural therapy techniques, Sarah learned to challenge her smoking-related thoughts and develop healthier coping mechanisms.

The workplace smoking cessation program also provided group support sessions during lunch breaks. Sarah connected with colleagues who were also on their quit journey, forming a supportive network. Sharing her struggles and celebrating milestones with others helped Sarah stay motivated and committed to her goal.

With the support of the smoking cessation service, Sarah successfully quit smoking after several months. She noticed immediate improvements in her physical fitness and experienced a renewed sense of vitality. The financial savings from not buying cigarettes allowed her to pursue new hobbies and activities that further enhanced her well-being.

Sarah's success story not only transformed her own life but also inspired her colleagues to consider quitting smoking. By sharing her experience and advocating for smoking cessation services, she created a positive ripple effect within her workplace, leading to a healthier and smoke-free environment for all.

6.4 The Impact of Success Stories

These success stories highlight the transformative impact that smoking cessation services can have on individuals' lives. They demonstrate that with the right support, motivation, and strategies, it is possible to overcome the challenges of nicotine addiction and achieve long-term abstinence.

Success stories not only inspire others to embark on their quit journey but also help reduce the stigma associated with quitting smoking. They showcase the diverse backgrounds and experiences of individuals who have successfully quit, illustrating that quitting is achievable for anyone, regardless of their circumstances.

By sharing these stories within communities, healthcare settings, and online platforms, we can create a supportive environment that encourages individuals to seek help and embark on their own path to a smoke-free life. Real-life experiences serve as beacons of hope, reminding us of the power of determination and the transformative impact of smoking cessation services.

In conclusion, success stories provide invaluable inspiration and encouragement to individuals considering quitting smoking. They showcase the effectiveness of smoking cessation services, demonstrate the wide-ranging benefits of quitting, and foster a sense of community among those on the quit journey. These stories serve as beacons of hope, empowering individuals to take control of their health and embrace a smoke-free life.

Chapter 7: Challenges and Solutions

7.1 Identifying Challenges

While smoking cessation services offer substantial benefits, they are not without challenges. It is essential to recognize and address these challenges to ensure the effectiveness and accessibility of these services.

One common challenge is the addiction to nicotine itself. Nicotine is a highly addictive substance, and individuals often struggle with intense cravings and withdrawal symptoms when attempting to quit. These challenges can lead to relapses and hinder the quitting process.

Another challenge is the social and environmental influences that promote smoking. Peer pressure, stress, and the availability of tobacco products can undermine an individual's motivation to quit. Additionally, individuals may face challenges in accessing smoking cessation services due to geographical barriers, financial constraints, or limited awareness of available resources.

7.2 Solutions and Strategies

To overcome these challenges, smoking cessation services employ a range of solutions and strategies that enhance the effectiveness and accessibility of support.

Comprehensive Support: Smoking cessation services provide comprehensive support that addresses the multifaceted nature of nicotine addiction. This includes combining behavioural interventions, pharmacotherapy, and ongoing counselling to address both the physical and psychological aspects of addiction. By employing a holistic approach, individuals have a higher likelihood of successfully quitting smoking.

Tailored Interventions: Recognizing that individuals have different needs and preferences, smoking cessation services offer tailored interventions. This includes personalized quit plans, individual counselling sessions, and the choice of various pharmacotherapy options. By addressing individual motivations, triggers, and challenges, tailored interventions increase the chances of success.

Education and Awareness: To tackle social and environmental influences, smoking cessation services prioritize education and awareness campaigns. By raising public awareness about the dangers of smoking, dispelling myths, and promoting the benefits of quitting, these campaigns aim to shift societal attitudes and norms. This helps create a supportive environment that encourages and facilitates quitting.

Community Engagement: Smoking cessation services actively engage with communities to ensure accessibility and address geographical and financial barriers. This involves partnerships with community organizations, local health departments, and employers to establish smoking cessation programs in various settings. By bringing support directly to the community, individuals have greater access to resources and assistance.

Technology and Digital Interventions: Embracing technology, smoking cessation services utilize digital interventions to expand their reach and accessibility. Online platforms, mobile applications, and virtual support groups provide convenient and immediate support to individuals. These platforms often offer self-help resources, tracking tools, and peer support, empowering individuals to quit smoking at their own pace.

Continuous Support: Quitting smoking is a journey, and ongoing support is crucial for long-term success. Smoking cessation services offer continuous support through follow-up sessions, support groups, and relapse prevention strategies.

By providing ongoing guidance, motivation, and reinforcement, individuals are better equipped to overcome challenges and maintain a smoke-free life.

7.3 Addressing Equity and Disparities

To ensure equitable access to smoking cessation services, it is vital to address disparities that exist among different populations. Efforts must be made to reach marginalized communities, low-income individuals, and groups with higher smoking prevalence. This includes tailoring interventions to cultural and socioeconomic contexts, providing language-appropriate resources, and addressing financial barriers through subsidized or free services.

Collaboration with healthcare providers, community leaders, and advocacy groups is essential in identifying and addressing disparities in smoking cessation services. By working together, stakeholders can develop targeted interventions, implement effective outreach strategies, and ensure that support reaches all individuals, regardless of their background or circumstances.

In conclusion, smoking cessation services face challenges related to nicotine addiction, social influences, and accessibility. However, through comprehensive support, tailored interventions, education, community engagement, and the use of technology, these challenges can be addressed. By prioritizing equity and working collaboratively, smoking cessation services can effectively support individuals in their journey towards quitting smoking and lead to a healthier, smoke-free society.

Chapter 8: Enhancing Smoking Cessation Services in the UK

8.1 Continuous Improvement

To ensure the ongoing effectiveness and impact of smoking cessation services in the UK, it is essential to focus on continuous improvement and innovation. By embracing new approaches, leveraging technology, and adapting to evolving needs, we can enhance the quality and reach of these services.

8.2 Integration and Collaboration

One key strategy for enhancing smoking cessation services is promoting integration and collaboration within the healthcare system. This involves fostering strong partnerships between smoking cessation specialists, primary care providers, hospitals, and community organizations. By integrating smoking cessation services into routine healthcare practices, individuals receive seamless support, and quitting smoking becomes a standard part of healthcare.

Collaboration with other sectors such as education, workplaces, and local government can also be instrumental in expanding the reach of smoking cessation services. By embedding support within educational curricula, implementing smoke-free policies in workplaces, and incorporating smoking cessation initiatives into public health campaigns, a comprehensive and multi-sectoral approach can be achieved.

8.3 Tailoring Services to Diverse Populations

To effectively address the needs of diverse populations, smoking cessation services should be tailored to be culturally sensitive and inclusive. This requires understanding the unique challenges faced by different communities, including ethnic minorities, LGBTQ+ individuals, individuals with mental health conditions, and pregnant women, among others.

Tailored interventions may involve providing language-appropriate resources, culturally relevant counselling, and support groups specific to certain populations. By acknowledging and addressing the diverse needs of individuals, smoking cessation services can ensure that all members of society have access to the support they need to quit smoking successfully.

8.4 Harnessing Technology and Digital Interventions

The advancement of technology presents significant opportunities to enhance smoking cessation services. Digital interventions, such as smartphone applications, online platforms, and telehealth services, can expand the reach and accessibility of support. These interventions provide self-help resources, interactive tools, remote counselling options, and personalized tracking systems, empowering individuals to quit smoking at their own pace.

Furthermore, utilizing data and analytics can help identify trends, evaluate program effectiveness, and make data-driven improvements to smoking cessation services.

By harnessing the power of technology, we can create innovative solutions that overcome barriers and improve the overall delivery of support.

8.5 Comprehensive Education and Awareness

Education and awareness campaigns are vital components of enhancing smoking cessation services. By raising public awareness about the risks of smoking, the benefits of quitting, and the availability of support services, we can encourage individuals to seek help and make informed decisions.

Comprehensive education should target various audiences, including schools, workplaces, healthcare settings, and community organizations. By equipping individuals with knowledge about the health consequences of smoking, the benefits of quitting, and the resources available, we can foster a society that supports and promotes smoking cessation.

8.6 Research and Evaluation

Continued research and evaluation are crucial for enhancing smoking cessation services in the UK. By conducting rigorous studies, monitoring outcomes, and evaluating program effectiveness, we can identify areas for improvement and implement evidence-based interventions.

Research can focus on identifying effective intervention methods, understanding barriers to quitting, exploring the impact of policy changes, and evaluating the long-term outcomes of smoking cessation programs.

This knowledge can inform policy decisions, guide resource allocation, and drive continuous improvement in smoking cessation services.

8.7 Policy Support

Supportive policies play a vital role in enhancing smoking cessation services. Governments and regulatory bodies can implement and enforce policies that promote smoke-free environments, increase tobacco taxation, and provide funding for smoking cessation programs. These policies create an environment that supports individuals in their quitting journey and reduces the prevalence of smoking within society.

In conclusion, enhancing smoking cessation services in the UK requires a multi-faceted approach. By focusing on continuous improvement, integration and collaboration, tailoring services to diverse populations, harnessing technology, promoting comprehensive education and awareness, conducting research and evaluation, and implementing supportive policies, we can strengthen the effectiveness and accessibility of these services. With these enhancements, we can create a society where quitting smoking is easier, support is readily available, and the overall health and well-being of individuals and communities are improved.

Chapter 9: Looking Ahead: Future Trends in Smoking Cessation

9.1 Advancements in Pharmacotherapy

Pharmacotherapy has been a cornerstone of smoking cessation services, and we can expect continued advancements in this field. Researchers are exploring new medications and delivery systems that target nicotine receptors more effectively, helping to reduce cravings and withdrawal symptoms. These innovations may provide additional options for individuals who have struggled to quit using traditional pharmacotherapy.

Furthermore, personalized medicine approaches may emerge, allowing healthcare providers to tailor medication choices based on an individual's genetic makeup and response to treatment. This precision medicine approach holds promise for optimizing the effectiveness of pharmacotherapy and increasing quit rates.

9.2 Digital Health Solutions

The integration of digital health solutions will continue to shape the landscape of smoking cessation services. Mobile applications, wearable devices, and virtual platforms will offer personalized support, tracking tools, and real-time feedback to individuals seeking to quit smoking.

These technologies can provide instant access to information, counselling, and support networks, empowering individuals to manage their quit journey anytime, anywhere.

Additionally, emerging technologies such as artificial intelligence and machine learning may be utilized to develop predictive models that identify personalized risk factors and tailor interventions accordingly. These intelligent systems have the potential to enhance the effectiveness and personalization of smoking cessation services.

9.3 Behavioural and Cognitive Approaches

Behavioural and cognitive approaches will continue to evolve, incorporating innovative strategies to address the psychological and behavioural aspects of smoking addiction. Cognitive behavioural therapy (CBT) techniques may be further refined, integrating virtual reality and immersive technologies to create realistic scenarios that help individuals develop coping mechanisms and resist smoking triggers.

Motivational interviewing, mindfulness-based interventions, and gamification techniques may also be incorporated into smoking cessation services, providing engaging and effective ways to support behaviour change and motivation.

9.4 Peer and Social Support Networks

Recognizing the power of social influence, future smoking cessation services will emphasize the role of peer support networks. Online communities, social media platforms, and virtual support groups will foster connections among individuals on their quit journey, enabling the sharing of experiences, encouragement, and motivation.

Community-based initiatives will also play a vital role, promoting social support within local neighbourhoods and workplaces. Collaborations between smoking cessation services and community organizations will create opportunities for collective efforts in reducing smoking prevalence and creating supportive environments.

9.5 Integration of Mental Health Support

Addressing the strong link between smoking and mental health, future smoking cessation services will integrate mental health support. Recognizing that individuals with mental health conditions face unique challenges when quitting smoking, these services will offer tailored interventions that address both smoking cessation and mental well-being.

Collaboration between smoking cessation specialists and mental health professionals will become more prevalent, ensuring that individuals receive comprehensive support that addresses the interconnected nature of smoking and mental health.

9.6 Global Initiatives and Policy Changes

The fight against smoking will continue on a global scale, with increased emphasis on policy changes and international collaboration. Governments worldwide will adopt stricter tobacco control measures, including plain packaging, increased taxation, and comprehensive advertising bans. These policy changes will create a less tobacco-friendly environment, making quitting more accessible and encouraging individuals to quit.

International cooperation will play a crucial role in sharing best practices, research findings, and successful strategies in smoking cessation.

Global initiatives will focus on reducing smoking-related health disparities, addressing the tobacco industry's influence, and advocating for smoke-free environments worldwide.

9.7 Continuous Research and Evaluation

To guide future advancements in smoking cessation services, continuous research and evaluation will be vital. Rigorous studies will investigate the effectiveness of emerging interventions, evaluate the long-term outcomes of different approaches, and assess the impact of policy changes.

Researchers will continue to explore the underlying mechanisms of nicotine addiction, identify new targets for intervention, and refine existing treatment modalities. This research will inform evidence-based practices and ensure that smoking cessation services remain at the forefront of scientific advancements.

In conclusion, the future of smoking cessation services holds promise for advancements in pharmacotherapy, digital health solutions, behavioural approaches, social support networks, mental health integration, global initiatives, and continuous research. By embracing these future trends, we can enhance the effectiveness, accessibility, and impact of smoking cessation services, ultimately leading to a healthier and smoke-free society.

Chapter 10: Conclusion: A Smoke-Free Future for the UK

The journey towards a smoke-free future in the UK is both an individual and collective effort. Smoking cessation services play a pivotal role in supporting individuals in their quest to quit smoking and achieving better health outcomes. Throughout this book, we have explored the importance of these services, the benefits they bring to individuals and society, the challenges they face, and the strategies employed to overcome those challenges.

By providing specialist smoking cessation advice and support, these services empower individuals to take control of their nicotine addiction, assess their readiness to quit, and work through the various aspects of their addiction. Through tailored interventions, comprehensive support, and continuous engagement, individuals are given the tools and resources necessary to embark on a successful quit journey.

We have seen how smoking cessation services offer significant benefits to society. By reducing smoking prevalence, these services contribute to improved public health outcomes, lower healthcare costs, and a decreased burden on the healthcare system. Moreover, a smoke-free society creates a healthier environment for all, reducing second-hand smoke exposure and improving the overall quality of life for individuals and communities.

Throughout this book, we have also highlighted the perspectives of specialists working in smoking cessation services. Their expertise, dedication, and commitment are essential in providing effective support and guidance to individuals seeking to quit smoking. Their role goes beyond just providing advice; they serve as motivators, educators, and compassionate supporters, working closely with clients to understand their unique needs and tailor interventions accordingly.

Furthermore, we have examined the importance of community settings and intervention methods in reaching individuals who may face geographical barriers, financial constraints, or limited awareness of available resources. By taking smoking cessation services directly to communities through partnerships with local organizations and workplaces, support becomes more accessible and inclusive.

Real-life success stories have demonstrated the transformative impact of smoking cessation services. These stories serve as powerful inspiration, highlighting that quitting smoking is achievable for anyone, regardless of their background or circumstances. They create a sense of hope, reduce stigma, and foster a supportive environment that encourages individuals to seek help and embark on their own quit journey.

However, smoking cessation services also face challenges.

Nicotine addiction, social influences, and accessibility barriers can hinder progress. Yet, we have explored the solutions and strategies employed to address these challenges. By continuously improving services, promoting integration and collaboration, tailoring interventions, harnessing technology, and implementing supportive policies, we can enhance the effectiveness and reach of smoking cessation services.

Looking ahead, we anticipate exciting future trends in smoking cessation services. Advancements in pharmacotherapy, the integration of digital health solutions, behavioural and cognitive approaches, peer and social support networks, and the integration of mental health support will shape the future landscape. Additionally, global initiatives, policy changes, and continuous research and evaluation will drive progress towards a smoke-free future.

In conclusion, a smoke-free future for the UK is within reach. With robust smoking cessation services, collective efforts, and ongoing dedication, we can empower individuals to quit smoking, improve public health, and create a society where smoking is a thing of the past. Together, we can build a healthier, smoke-free future for the UK, benefiting individuals, communities, and generations to come.

References:

1. Action on Smoking and Health (ASH). (2021). Smoking statistics: UK. Retrieved from https://ash.org.uk/information-and-resources/fact-sheets/statistics/

2. Bauld, L., Hiscock, R., Dobbie, F., Aveyard, P., Coleman, T., Leonardi-Bee, J., ... & McRobbie, H. (2020). English stop-smoking services: One-year outcomes. International Journal of Environmental Research and Public Health, 17(8), 2726.

3. Fiore, M. C., Jaén, C. R., Baker, T. B., Bailey, W. C., Benowitz, N. L., Curry, S. J., ... & Wewers, M. E. (2008). Treating tobacco use and dependence: 2008 update. Clinical Practice Guideline. US Department of Health and Human Services.

4. McEwen, A., West, R., McRobbie, H., & Hajek, P. (2020). Manual of Smoking Cessation: A Guide for Counsellors and Practitioners. Wiley.

5. National Institute for Health and Care Excellence (NICE). (2018). Stop smoking interventions and services. Retrieved from https://www.nice.org.uk/guidance/ph10

6. Office for National Statistics (ONS). (2021). Smoking habits in the UK: 2021. Retrieved from https://www.ons.gov.uk/peoplepopulationandcommunity/healthandsocialcare/healthandlifeexpectancies/bulletins/adultsmokinghabitsingreatbritain/2021

7. Public Health England (PHE). (2020). Local stop smoking services: Service delivery and monitoring guidance 2020/21. Retrieved from https://assets.publishing.service.gov.uk/governme nt/uploads/system/uploads/attachment_data/file/ 862834/Local_stop_smoking_services_service_deli very_and_monitoring_guidance_2020_to_2021.pdf

8. World Health Organization (WHO). (2021). Tobacco. Retrieved from https://www.who.int/news-room/fact-sheets/detail/tobacco

www.ingramcontent.com/pod-product-compliance
Lightning Source LLC
Chambersburg PA
CBHW062302290526
45794CB00006B/2663